Six Pack Abs: How to Get Ripped Abs

The Truth on How to Reveal Your Six Pack Abs With Diet and Exercise

Kelly Larson

Copyright Act of 1976, the scanning, uploading and electronic sharing of any part of this book without the explicit written consent or permission of the publisher constitutes unlawful piracy and the theft of intellectual property.

If you would like to use material or content from this book (other than for review purposes), prior written permission must be obtained from the publisher.

You can contact the publishing company at admin@speedypublishing.com. Thank you for not infringing on the author's rights.

Speedy Publishing LLC (c) 2014
40 E. Main St., #1156
Newark, DE 19711
www.speedypublishing.co

Ordering Information:
Quantity sales; Special discounts are available on quantity purchases by corporations, associations, and others. For details, contact the "Special Sales Department" at the address above.

This is a reprint book.

Manufactured in the United States of America

Table of Contents

Publisher's Notes i

Chapter 1: Introduction 1

Chapter 2: Are Visible Abs Even Possible? 4

Chapter 3: Have Realistic Expectations When Training for Abs 6

Chapter 4: Nutrition and Diet Musts for Six Pack Abs 9

Chapter 5: 5 Super Foods for Six Pack Abs 13

Chapter 6: Supplements to Use in Your Quest for Six Pack Abs 16

Chapter 7: 5 Ab Exercises that Work 19

Chapter 8: Cardio and Six Pack Abs 22

Chapter 9: Ab Workout Walk Through 24

Chapter 10: Pitfalls to Avoid 27

Chapter 11: Maintaining Your Abs Year Round 30

Chapter 12: Take Action and Begin Your Six Pack Ab Training Today 33

Meet the Author 36

More Books by Kelly Larson 37

Publisher's Notes

Disclaimer

This publication is intended to provide helpful and informative material. It is not intended to diagnose, treat, cure, or prevent any health problem or condition, nor is intended to replace the advice of a physician. No action should be taken solely on the contents of this book. Always consult your physician or qualified health-care professional on any matters regarding your health and before adopting any suggestions in this book or drawing inferences from it.

The author and publisher specifically disclaim all responsibility for any liability, loss or risk, personal or otherwise, which is incurred as a consequence, directly or indirectly, from the use or application of any contents of this book.

Any and all product names referenced within this book are the trademarks of their respective owners. None of these owners have sponsored, authorized, endorsed, or approved this book.

Always read all information provided by the manufacturers' product labels before using their products. The author and publisher are not responsible for claims made by manufacturers.

Print Edition 2014

Chapter 1: Introduction

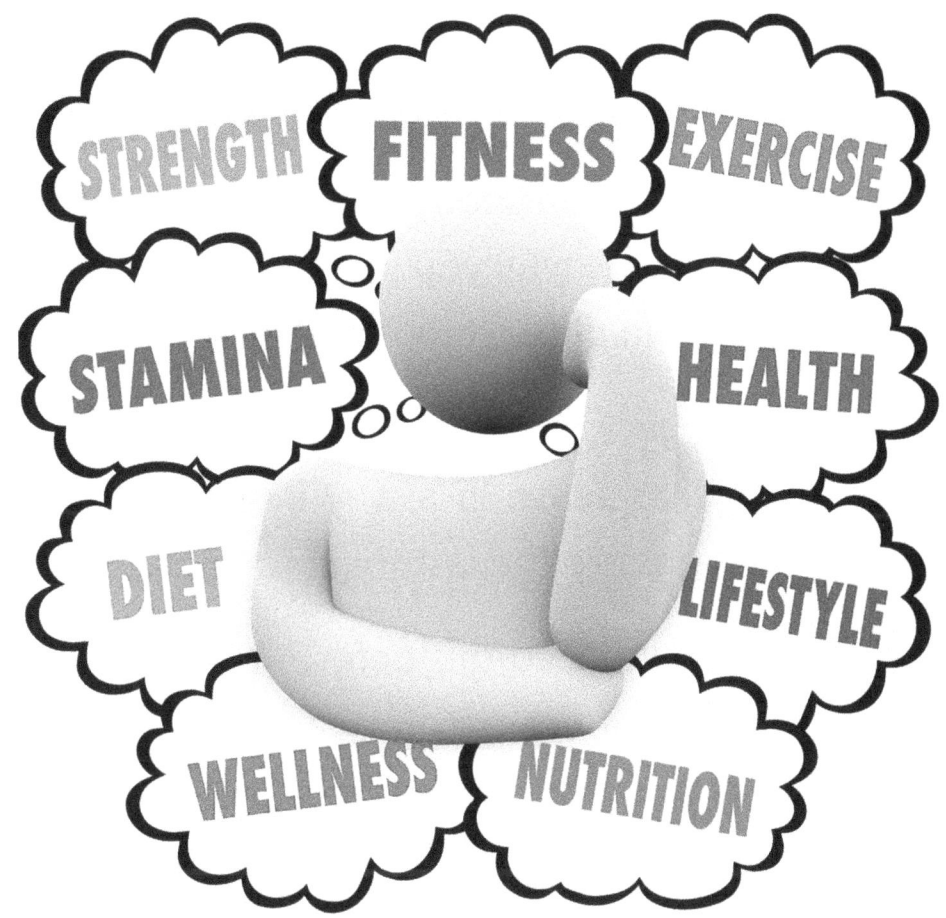

Six pack abs seems to be the magical unicorn that so many people are chasing after but never seem to catch.

Many people wonder why they don't have six pack abs. That question is a bit confusing however because in truth we all have abs. Of course having abs and having a six pack are obviously two very different things in some people's mind.

The truth of the matter is we all have the same abdominal muscles. What we do with them, how we work them and how we try to define them is up to us.

Every single person has a six pack, just the same as every single person has a pair of biceps. The shape and definition of your six pack is dependent on many factors just like the shape and size of your biceps.

Unfortunately your genetics is not something that you can change. You can't change your body type any more than you can change your height. That is why you see that having visible abs is easy for some people and difficult for others.

To many people a six pack is the ultimate goal when it comes to working out. This makes sense in a way because whenever you are losing weight the abs are the last thing to appear.

You have probably experienced this before. You are trying to lose weight and you notice differences in your shoulders and arms, but nothing really in your abs. That is because when you lose fat your body works from the outside in. That is why the abs are so hard to uncover.

You have to realize that your body doesn't care about how you look. Your body is only interested in survival. Your body doesn't think that single digit body fat is a good idea, so it takes work and determination. However that can be said of anything worth having.

The bottom line is that everyone has abs. The reason that everyone doesn't have visible abs depends on a variety of factors. For some people it is genetic, for other people it is lack of consistent effort, or simply not wanting to change. However, no matter what anyone says or tries to tell you, you do have abs, now it's up to you and the help of this guide to transform them into a six pack. Whether or not you put in the work, and take the time to reveal it is up to you.

Chapter 2: Are Visible Abs Even Possible?

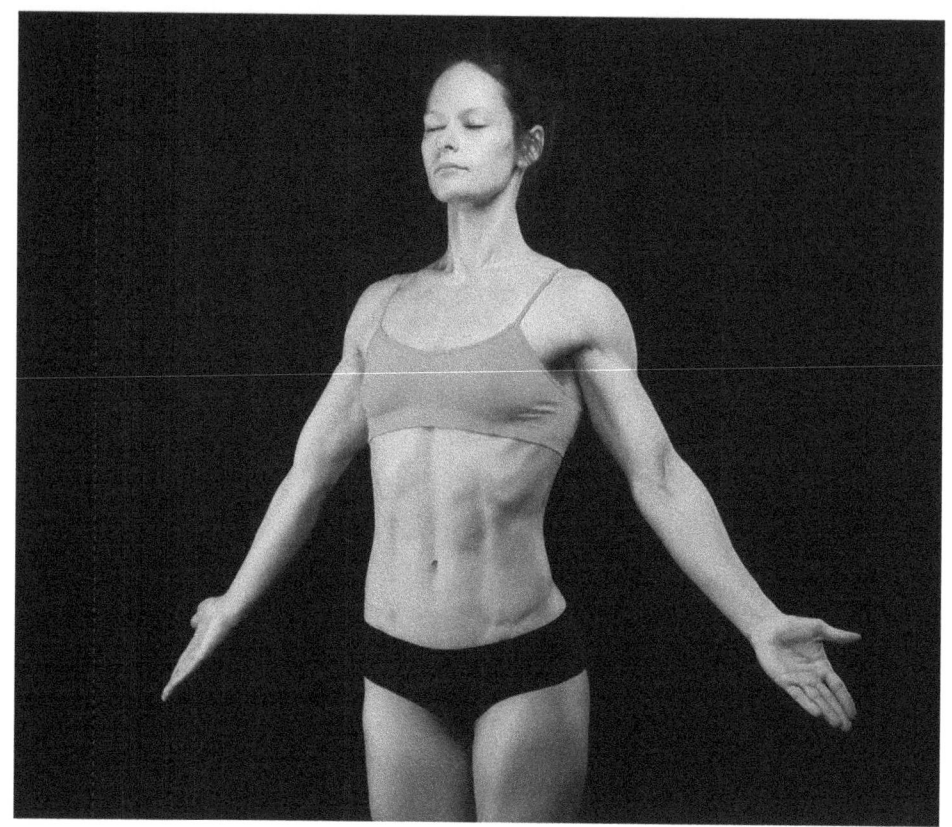

With all the products out there promoting six pack abs it is obvious that a lot of people need help.

The majority of people struggle with it so much that many people just give up and think that it is impossible. One thing you have to realize is that in order for you to have a visible six pack you have to reach a certain body fat percentage.

You can increase the visual appeal of your abs by doing ab work and building the muscles. However, if you are still carrying too much body fat they will not be well defined.

So in order to have visible abs you have to reduce body fat. This is easier for some people than others, but everyone can do it. There are many factors that go into weight loss. Calories consumed and calories burned are just a small part of it. You also have to consider your genetics, body type, and hormonal interaction.

All of these factors can add up and complicate the process. People either get overwhelmed by all the different aspects, or they completely overlook some of them. Either way this can make it seem like building a six pack is impossible.

You can feel like you are doing everything right. You can be eating perfectly, you can be training well, and some other hidden factor can be slowing you down.

Sometimes simple things such as stress or lack of sleep can throw your hormones out of balance and cause you to retain water. The water you retain can hide the progress you are making, and you start to get frustrated. Once you get frustrated you get more stressed, and it can become a vicious cycle.

However, the truth is that everyone can develop their abs. The main variable is how long it will take. Some people always seem to have abs no matter what they do or eat. For other people it is going to take a lot of work, and it is going to be frustrating. Like with most anything else training related, consistency is the key to success. If you stay consistent and monitor all the aspects of your training, life, and environment then you can build an awesome set of visible abs.

Chapter 3: Have Realistic Expectations When Training for Abs

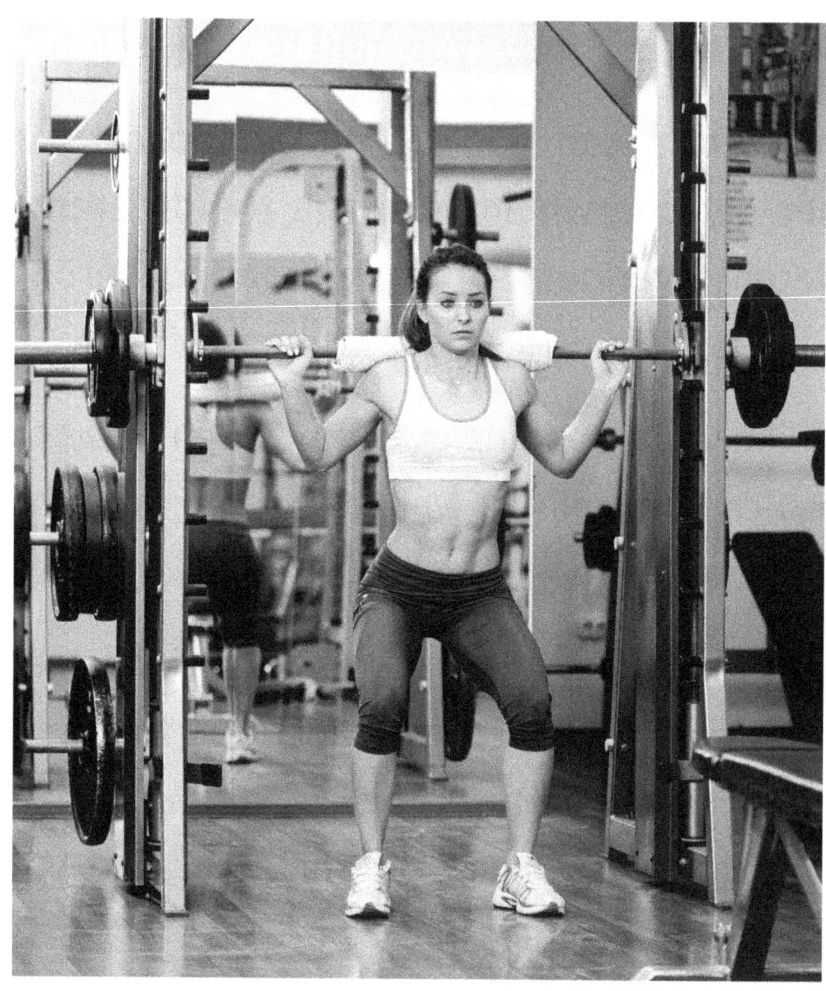

Training your abs is no different than training any other muscle. If you want results you have to have a plan and you have to put forth consistent effort.

Another thing to consider with ab training is that you have to be patient. The abs are always the last thing to reveal themselves, so it makes sense that they will take the most time to develop.

3 Things to Consider When Beginning Ab Training

- It's going to take longer than you expect.
- It's going to be harder than you thought.
- You are going to have to diet.

It cannot be overemphasized that getting a six pack is really hard work. The problem is there are so many infomercials out there that tell you that you can have a six pack in eight weeks. And even though you know that isn't likely it is hard to resist the temptation to believe it. We all fall victim to such promises, and when we constantly see these types of ads it is hard not to have an unrealistic expectation on how long it will take.

The problem is that when you set unrealistic expectations, chances are you will fail. And when you fail to reach your goal in the time you decided you are likely to get frustrated and give up. Once you give up the first time it gets harder and harder to start again because you don't expect it to work.

This happens in all areas of fitness, but seems to happen the most when it comes to building a six pack. The reason is that having a six pack is directly tied to your body fat percentage. You cannot have a six pack with a high level of body fat, so diet is always a major factor.

People are constantly going on diets for a few weeks, not dropping weight as fast as they want, and ultimately quitting. The yo-yo diet syndrome is definitely something that you want to avoid. Besides the time factor, another thing to consider is lower back training. As with all your training you want to make sure your physique is balanced. If you significantly increase your ab training without increasing your lower back training then you will develop muscular imbalances. This is a recipe for disaster and can lead to lower back issues or injury. Take this into consideration when you plan your training.

The bottom line is before you have any visions of washboard abs and start to train abs, be realistic about how long it is going to take and balance out your training. Just realize it is going to take longer than you want, and it is going to be more work than you want to do. However, the pay-off will be worth it!

Once you reach your goal you will have a sense of accomplishment, and an awesome six pack too.

Chapter 4: Nutrition and Diet Musts for Six Pack Abs

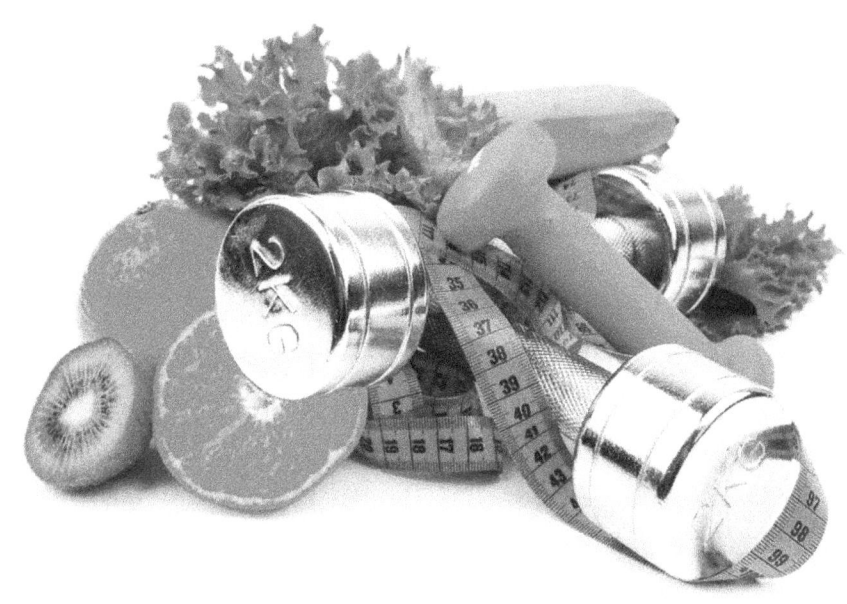

As important as training is, when it comes to abs, diet is more important.

No other muscle group is as dependent on diet as the abs, because abs take a certain body fat percentage to appear. While it is true that you can build the abs to be more visible, you still are going to have to drop body fat to have a six pack.

In this part we are going to look at five nutrition tips for six pack abs:

- Eliminate Sugar
- Increase Protein Consumption
- Eat Healthy Fats

- Eat Whole Unprocessed Foods
- Drinks Lots of Water

Eliminate Sugar – Pretty much every piece of diet advice will tell you to reduce or eliminate sugar intake. This list is obviously no exception. The main problem with sugar is that it causes an insulin spike.

Once insulin is present all fat burning comes to a halt. If you want your body to be a fat burning machine then you have to keep blood sugar levels steady and reduce the effects of insulin. That is not to say that you have to avoid carbs altogether. A quality post workout shake with carbs in it is a good way to replenish glycogen in the muscle and help you recover.

Increase Protein Consumption – While you do need a caloric deficit to lose weight you don't want to lose the muscle you have built.

If you are lowering carb intake then you have to get those calories from somewhere else. Consuming protein in the form of lean cuts of meat is optimal. Protein shakes are convenient, but it is better to get most of your calories from whole foods. Drinking your calories does not give you the same level of satisfaction, and being in a caloric deficit is hard enough. Also there is a thermogenic effect of digesting foods that you do not get when you drink your calories.

Eat Healthy Fats – No matter what you may hear, low fat diets are ineffective. Your body needs good healthy fats.

You also have to consider that the more fat that you consume the more efficient you become at processing it. If you reduce your fat intake then your body does not produce as many fat burning enzymes. So you should include healthy fats in your meal plans. Just pay attention to your calories as fats are very calorie dense.

Eat Whole Unprocessed Foods – This is good advice whether you want abs or not. Both from a health standpoint and from a dieting standpoint it is best to consume unprocessed foods. These foods have more nutritional value, and when you are reducing calories you need the most nutrient dense foods you can find.

Drinks Lots of Water – Hydration is important whether you are dieting or not. However, when you are dieting it can help for numerous reasons. Drinking lots of water helps you to feel full and reduces hunger cravings. It is a fact that the more water that you drink, the more water that you excrete. You can reduce your water retention by drinking more water, and the less water you retain the more visible your abs are.

None of these suggestions are particularly exciting. In fact you will probably find these on every diet tips list you ever read. There is a reason for that; they work. People are always looking for short cuts to dieting and getting abs, but short cuts are worthless if you don't cover the basics first. If you cover the basics on this list first you will make your ab training that much more effective, and you'll see your abs sooner.

CHAPTER 5: 5 SUPER FOODS FOR SIX PACK ABS

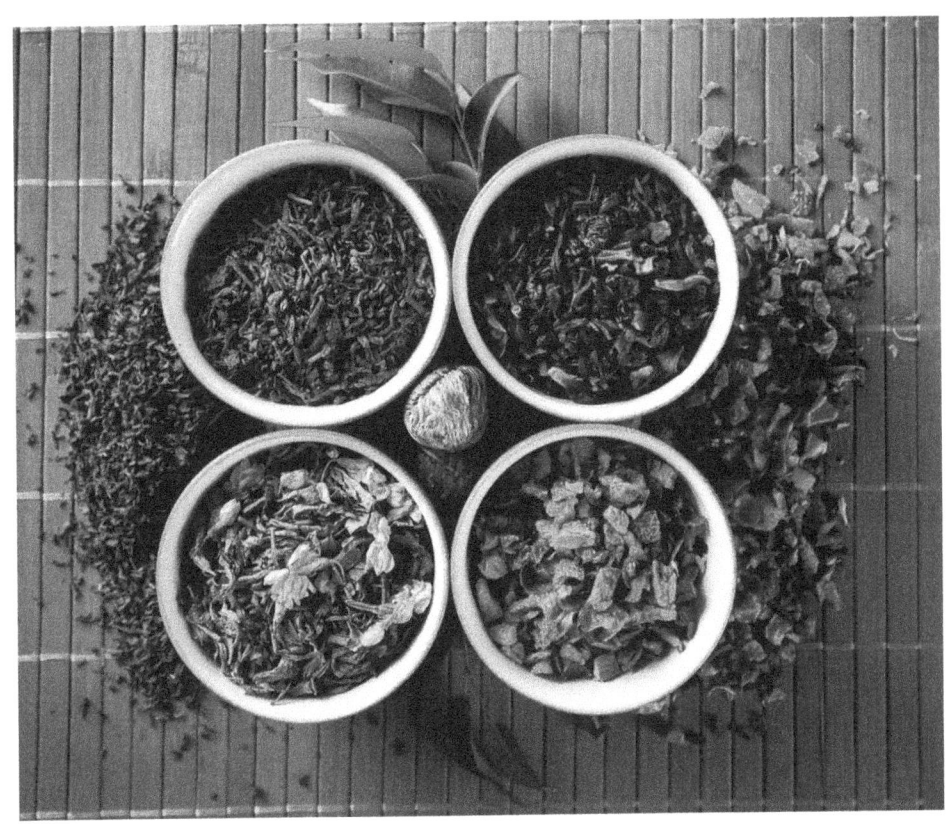

There are a lot of factors when it comes to building six pack abs. Some of them, like genetics, are beyond your control. However, training and diet are two things you can control.

Make no mistake about it ab training is very important. However, your dream of abs lives and dies with your diet.

You can do all the work you want in the gym, and completely sabotage your results in the kitchen. Since abs are the last to appear and the first to disappear diet will always play a huge part in how your six pack looks.

How restrictive you have to be with in regards to diet depends on many things. However, just when you might start to think it is impossible to get your six pack there is good news. There are actually super foods that can help speed up the fat loss process and bring your abs out for the entire world to see.

5 Super Foods For Six Pack Abs

- Whole Eggs
- Grass Fed Butter
- Grass Fed Beef
- Wild Fish
- Dark Leafy Greens

Whole Eggs – You might not expect eggs to be on this list but they are an excellent source of protein. They have a very impressive amino acid profile, and they offer good fats. Eggs will not only help with fat loss, but they will help you build muscle. This is a one-two punch when it comes to building a six pack. It is important to note that when it comes to eggs you should be eating free range organic.

Grass Fed Butter – I am sure you think that butter will make you fat. The truth it is depends on the type of butter. Grass fed butter is one of the best sources of conjugated linoleic acid (CLA). CLA has been shown to not only help with weight loss, but increase your resistance to carcinogens. Not only that, but it has a great ration of Omega 3 to Omega 6 fatty acids.

Grass Fed Beef – Much like butter, grass fed beef has many more health benefits than your average ground beef. It has been shown to have 10 times the beta-carotene, three times the Vitamin E and 3 times the Omega 3 fatty acids.

Wild Fish – We all know that fish oil is a powerful supplement, and that we eat far too much Omega 6 and not enough Omega 3. Wild caught fish are full of healthy Omega-3's as well as being high in protein.

Dark Leafy Greens – We all know we need to eat more vegetables, but when it comes to six pack abs Popeye was right. Dark leafy greens such as spinach, kale, and bok choy are perfect super foods for your six pack plans. They help you reach your nutritional requirements, and a great source of vitamins and minerals, and have very few calories. They are nutrient dense foods and when you are dieting that is a necessity.

I hope this list of superfoods helps in your awareness of super foods that can have a big impact on your diet and in revealing those six pack abs.

Chapter 6: Supplements to Use in Your Quest for Six Pack Abs

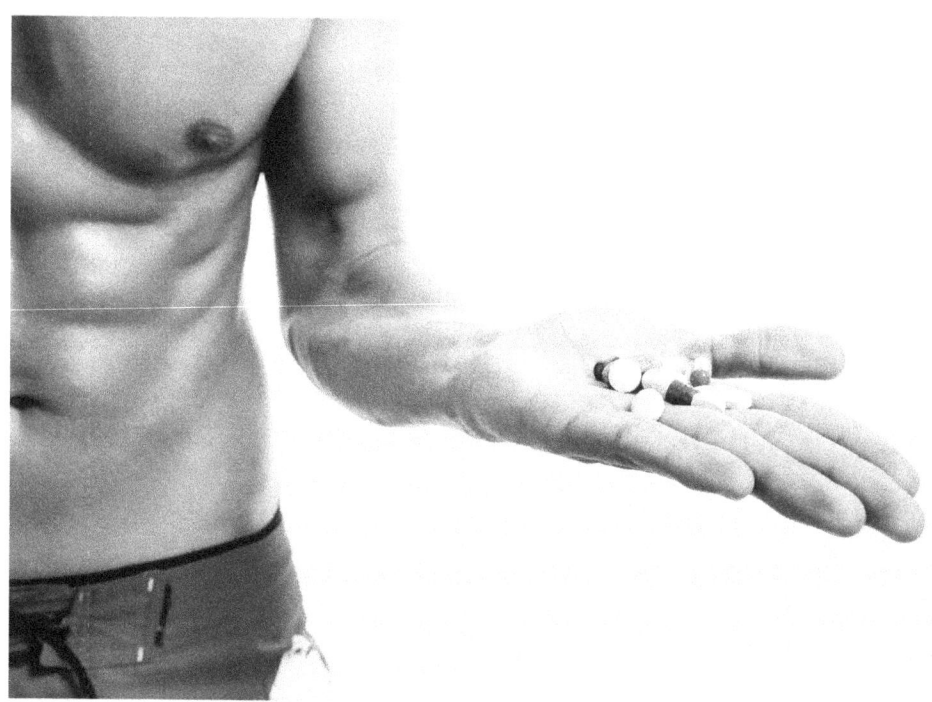

We cannot get away from the fact that diet has a huge impact on our quest for six pack abs. What you eat has a huge impact on your results.

The supplement industry knows this, and makes billions of dollars each year selling you quick fix solutions to your problems. Unfortunately most of the supplements out there are nothing more than snake oil. They are here today, gone tomorrow, and when they leave, they take your hard earned money with them.

The best supplements are the ones that have stood the test of time. People spend too much time looking for the latest and greatest shortcut. The truth is if you want six pack abs you are going to have to work for it, and it is going to take longer than you want. To help speed up the process though here are some solid supplement choices.

5 Best Supplements for Six Pack Abs

- Caffeine
- CLA
- Yohimbe
- Synephrine
- Green Tea

Caffeine – Not only does your morning coffee help you wake up in the morning; it aids in fat loss. Caffeine is a CNS stimulant that binds to fat and enhances fat burning. Unfortunately your body can become immune to your normal caffeine dose so it may be necessary to cycle on and off from time to time to get the same effect.

CLA – Conjugated linoleic acid is a healthy fat that is a true powerhouse when it comes to six pack abs. It has been shown to boost strength, shred body fat and build muscle. CLA actually blocks certain fat storing enzymes, thus preventing the storage of fat.

Yohimbe – You will find Yohimbe in most fat burning stacks. Its effects are well documented. It works in a different method from other fat burnings in that it blacks the alpha receptors on fat cells. Yohimbe can be taken orally, or if you find it in a cream form you can apply it directly to the ab area.

Synephrine – We all know the caffeine, ephedrine and aspirin stack worked well for fat loss. Unfortunately ephedrine is no longer available. Synephrine has a similar chemical structure to ephedrine, but it increases fat burning without increasing your heart rate or raising your blood pressure.

Green Tea – Green tea contains catechins. EGCG is the main catechin, and it is responsible for the thermogenic effects of green tea. EGCG works to inhibit norepinephrine break down, which allows you to maintain a high level of calorie burning.

This might not be an exciting list, but the truth is these supplements work.

You can waste your time with the latest and greatest, or you can stick to the basics. There is a reason these supplements have been around forever. Add them to your mix and you will see an increase in your results.

CHAPTER 7: 5 AB EXERCISES THAT WORK

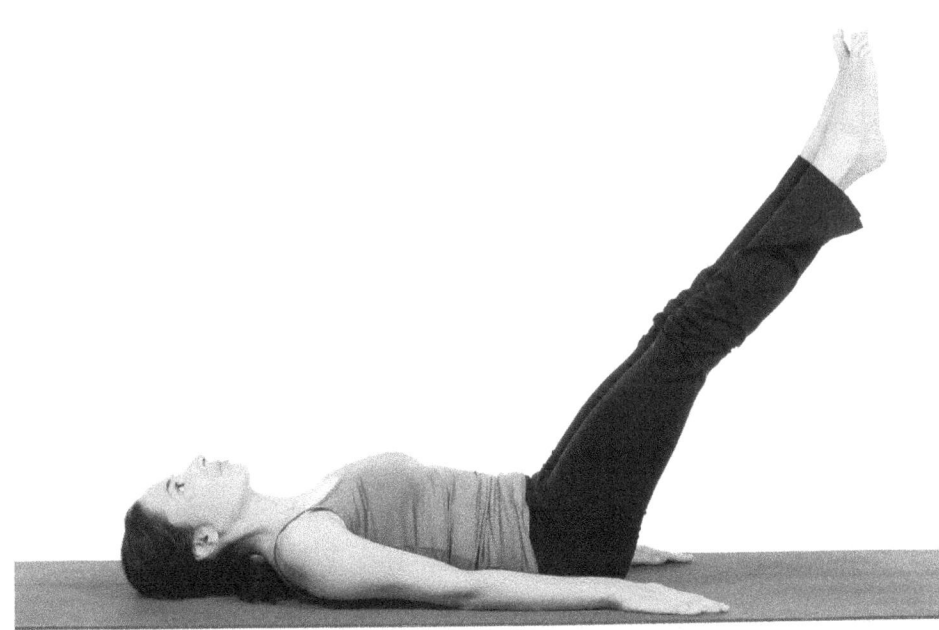

For many people ab training just means lying on the floor and doing crunches. They think that if they just do 1000 crunches a day they will have 6 pack abs in 8 weeks.

Who can blame them since they are constantly shown commercials for workouts promising just that?

Unfortunately we all know that is not true. To really build a six pack you have to mix up your exercises and hit the abs from different angles.

Top 5 Ab Exercises

- Standing Cable Pulldown
- Ab wheel
- Bicycle Crunches
- Reverse Crunches
- Leg Raises

Standing Cable Pulldown – One thing people seem to forget is that the abs are muscles. They respond to weighted training as well. The standing cable pulldown is an excellent way to add some weight into your ab training. It also works your abs while standing which is important if you are an athlete.

Ab wheel – Before there were planks there was the ab wheel. This is one of best toys you can buy for the gym. It hits the abs just as hard as planks, and allows you to do all kinds of variations. Even better news is that they are relatively inexpensive and can fit in your gym bag.

Bicycle Crunches – Often times when it comes to ab training we only work in one plane. However the abs are built to perform in numerous planes. Adding some twisting to your ab exercises is a great way to stimulate new muscles like the oblique and serratus.

Reverse Crunches – We spend so much time focusing on the upper abs that we often forget about the lower abs. This imbalance can cause a number of problems. Besides building a midsection that is not symmetrical you are setting yourself up for an injury. While ab muscles are very resistant to injury, if you happen to pull one you will remember it forever.

Leg Raises – This is one of the best lower ab exercises there is. You can do this is a variety of ways. You can use a chin-up bar or a roman chair; you can do them with straight or bent legs a well. Whichever combination that you choose to use just be consistent in doing them. They really will help round out your ab development.

This is just a short list of ab exercises to help add some variety to your training. If you need any help with how to perform the exercise or technique, just perform a search on Google and you will find a whole array of descriptions, demonstrations and variations.

Don't get stuck in the rut of thinking that crunches are the only thing you can do. You have to mix it up in order to keep your body growing. Don't let your progress stagnate or allow yourself to get bored. If you stick with it you will eventually reach your six pack goals.

CHAPTER 8: CARDIO AND SIX PACK ABS

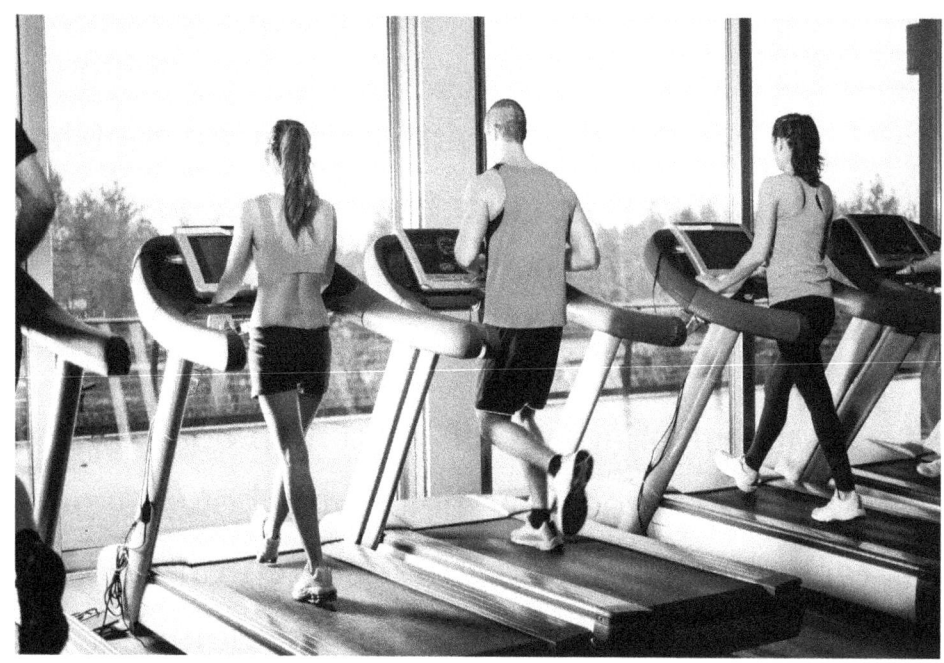

For some reason when people want six pack abs the first thing they think is that they just need to do a little more cardio and they will get there. Obviously diet and other training aspects factor into the equation. Cardio does have its place in your six pack ab training; you just have to be careful not to overdo it.

Some people can become obsessed with getting their six pack, which isn't necessarily bad. However, when that obsession leads to them doing hours and hours of cardio a week it can be a problem.

When you put yourself in too great of a caloric deficit your body will have no choice but to burn muscle. While you will be losing weight, that weight will be muscle and you continue to get softer and softer.

When it comes to cardio for your six pack less is often better if your diet and training are on point then you don't need to go crazy with your cardio. In fact if your cardio is intense enough you could get away with doing only an hour a week or so.

HIIT Cardio for Six Pack Abs

If you have never heard of HIIT it stands for high intensity interval training. It consists of doing a short duration of really intense exercise followed by a longer duration of lower intensity exercise. For the sake of cardio it might involve sprinting for 20-30 seconds and then walking for 90 seconds to 2 minutes. Or sprinting on a bike or rowing machine or whatever form of cardio that you can out all out effort into and then have a rest period.

HIIT cardio is the best bet cardio for fat loss. With HIIT you hit your muscles hard with short, intense workouts that burn the maximal amount of fat. Not only that, but you continue to burn fat after your workout, and at a much higher rate than traditional slow steady cardio. A couple of HIIT sessions a week is all you need. It is much more effective and efficient than spending 45 minutes a day on a treadmill.

CHAPTER 9: AB WORKOUT WALK THROUGH

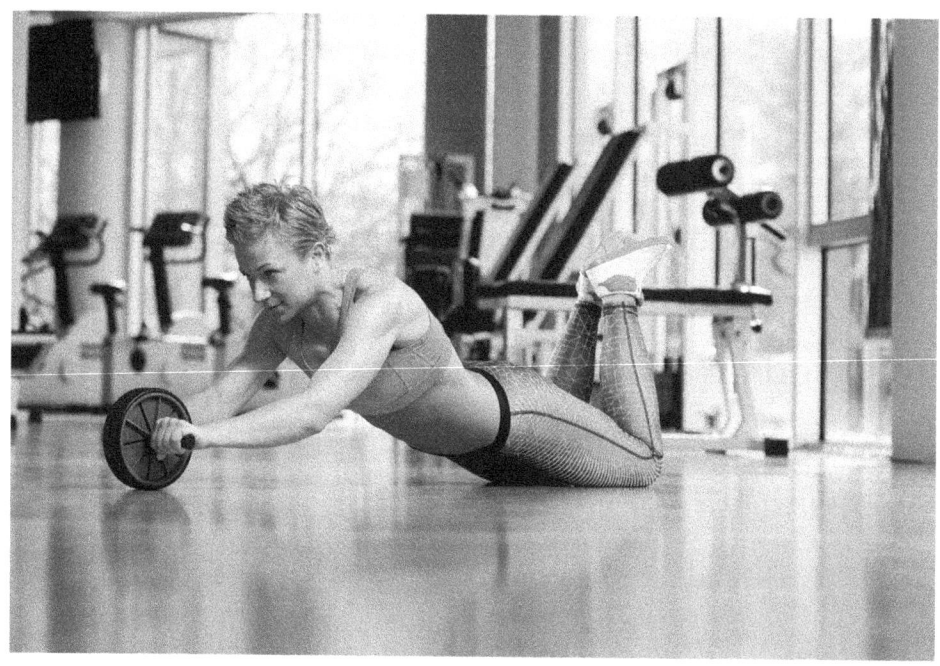

So you are ready to start your journey towards six pack abs. The problem is you have no idea what you should do. Here is a sample routine that is a good place to start. Remember it is important when you are just starting out to learn proper exercise technique. Any bad habits you learn in the beginning will tend to stick with you, so remember if you need help just Google the exercise and lots of options will become available to you.

Beginner's Ab Workout

- Cable Ab Pulldown 3 X 15 (add weight)
- Straight Leg Raises 3 X 15
- Hyperextension Side Bends 3X 10-15 (add weight)
- Ab Wheel 2 X 20

Cable Ab Pulldown – This is one of the best ab exercises because it allows you to use weight, and to train the abs while standing.

Lying on the ground and training you abs is very unnatural, you need to learn to contract your abs while standing. For this exercise you need a cable machine with a high pulley and a triceps rope.

Take a normal athletic stance face away from the machine. Take the handles and pull them down around the back of your neck so you can hold them against your chest. From there you perform a standing crunch until your upper body is perpendicular to the floor; then return to an upright position.

Straight Leg Raises – Grab a high bar and just hang until all the momentum goes away.

From there you flex your entire body, especially your lats and abs. With your legs straight begin to lift them. Your goal is to get your feet to the bar, but you may need to work up to that. At the very least you should bring your legs to parallel to the floor. Lower your legs and repeat.

Hyperextension Side Bends – On a 45 degree hyperextension bench, begin by standing sideways. Make sure the pad is properly placed against your hip, and lower yourself down towards the floor.

When your upper body is parallel to the floor flex your obliques hard as you return to your starting position. This is an exercise that you can add weight to by using a dumbbell in the hand closest to the floor, a weight plate against your chest, or a weight plate behind your head.

Ab Wheel – This basic exercise is often overlooked, but it is very effective. It is basically an ab plank with movement added.

Simply kneel on the floor, and grip the handles of the wheel in front of you. Slowly roll out as far as you can, and then contract your abs as you return to the starting position. Once you have gotten the hang of it you can roll out to either side instead of just a straight line for added variety.

Chances are if you are consistent you will quickly out grow this workout. However, when you are just starting out it is always a good idea to keep it simple. Obviously there are many more advanced techniques that you will learn as your progress, but this routine is a good place for you to start.

CHAPTER 10: PITFALLS TO AVOID

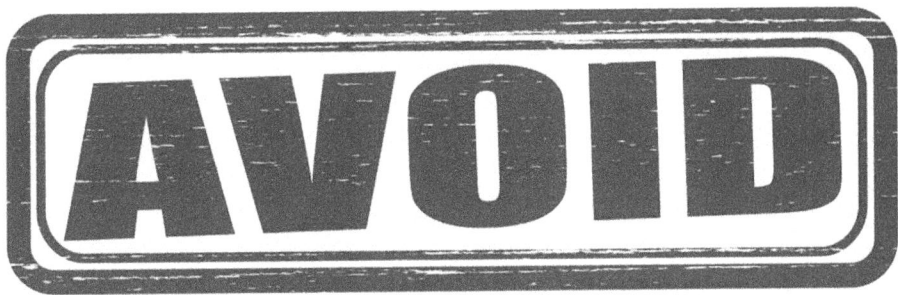

So many people want six pack abs, but very few people have them. Have you ever wondered why that is? The truth is that many people train their abs incorrectly, and get poor results. Those poor results lead to them giving up. So how can you avoid making the same mistakes that they are making?

Top 5 Ab Training Mistakes

- Doing Too Many Crunches
- Not Enough Intensity
- Not Actually Training Abs
- Only Training Upper Abs
- Trying to Out Crunch a Poor Diet

Doing Too Many Crunches – Crunches are a great exercise for six pack abs, but they aren't the only exercise. Too often people fall into the trap of just doing crunches, and obviously this is far from optimal. Your abs are made up of numerous different muscles, they move in different direction, and in different planes. You have to constantly hit them from different angles to get results.

Not Enough Intensity – For some reason people think that high reps are the only way to train abs. This simply is not true.

Your abs respond to training just like any other training, and constantly doing sets of 50 is not always the best way to go. You need to vary your intensity of your ab work just like you would any other muscle group. In fact you should focus on training to grow your abs instead of just toning them. It is almost impossible for your abs to get too big, so mix in some intensity techniques and get them growing.

Not Actually Training Abs – This actually happens more than you might think. Some people think that they can just diet and cardio their way to a six pack.

Other people try to work their abs, but miss the mark. They end of spending the majority of their ab workout hitting their hip flexors and aggravating their spinal erectors. If you want six pack abs you have to actually train your abs, and you have to train them correctly.

Only Training Upper Abs – This is similar to the above mentioned mistake. You have to understand that the abs consist of much more than just the upper rectus abdominis. The truth is there are

4 ab areas to train.

The other 3 include the lower rectus abdominis, the obliques, and the transverse abdominis. When you train your abs and only hit the upper abs it is similar to training your arms and only doing biceps. For complete development you have to hit all the ab muscles.

Trying to Out Crunch a Poor Diet – This is one that many people fall prey to. They think that they can have a bad diet, and if they just work hard enough they will still have a six pack. Unfortunately this just isn't true. There is a saying that you can't out train a bad diet, and it is very true. Yes you build your abs in the gym, but you remove the fat that is covering them in the kitchen.

While there is more mistakes that can be made when it comes to ab training, these seem to be the most common. If you concentrate on avoiding them your ab training will be well ahead of the game. With consistent, intelligent ab training you can get the six pack you want.

Chapter 11: Maintaining Your Abs Year Round

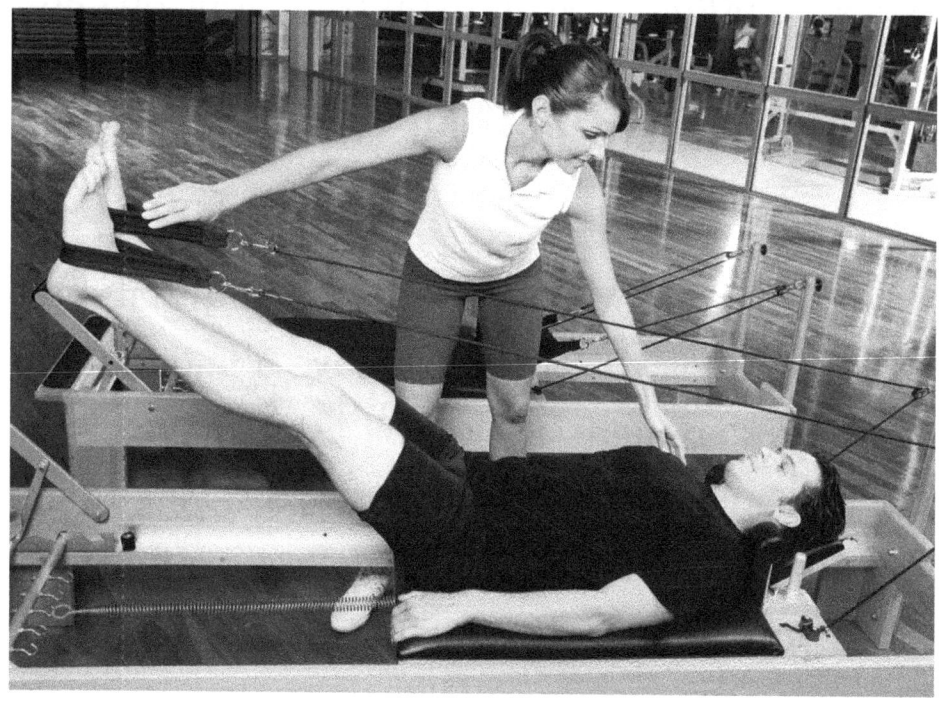

If you are one of the few people that have built an impressive set of abs you now face an even bigger challenge. How do I maintain my six pack year round? Thankfully ab maintenance is slightly easier than digging them out from underneath the fat to begin with...but not by much.

Society is always trying to sabotage your results with poor food choices or excuses to skip the gym altogether. Here are some tips to help you keep your abs all year.

5 Tips to Maintaining Six Pack Abs

- Make Smart Decisions
- Be Prepared

- Avoid Stress
- Schedule Cheat Days
- Work for Your Carbs

Make Smart Decisions – This can apply to any goal that you have, but when it comes to abs you have to understand that every choice has a consequence. Usually it comes down to food choices, but this can also apply to skipping a training day. You have to ask yourself if the decision you are about to make gets you closer to your goals or not.

Be Prepared – Whenever you are away from your own kitchen poor food choices are waiting to surprise you. Social gatherings and peer pressure are a great way for you to lose your abs. So always have healthy alternatives available.

Avoid Stress – We all know that stress causes cortisol to be released into your bloodstream. If your cortisol levels are constantly elevated it will stimulate fat storage. This obviously is a death sentence for your abs, so try to avoid stress at all costs.

Schedule Cheat Days – When trying to maintain your abs you are going to always have to watch what you eat. Over the course of a year that can lead up to a lot of frustration. So rather than risk getting fed up and binging it is best to schedule cheat days. This means you always have something to look forward to.

Work for Your Carbs – We all love carbs, but the insulin response they cause can wreak havoc on our abs. You don't have to deprive yourself of them, but you should always make sure you earn them. Make sure you are consistently burning enough calories to warrant eating them.

One thing you must realize is that your body doesn't care if your abs are visible. In fact it would prefer it if you carried an extra layer of fat to help ensure survival. To maintain abs year round you are going to have to have a plan, and stick to it. You can allow yourself an occasional liberty, but if you ease up too much your abs will go back into hiding.

Chapter 12: Take Action and Begin Your Six Pack Ab Training Today

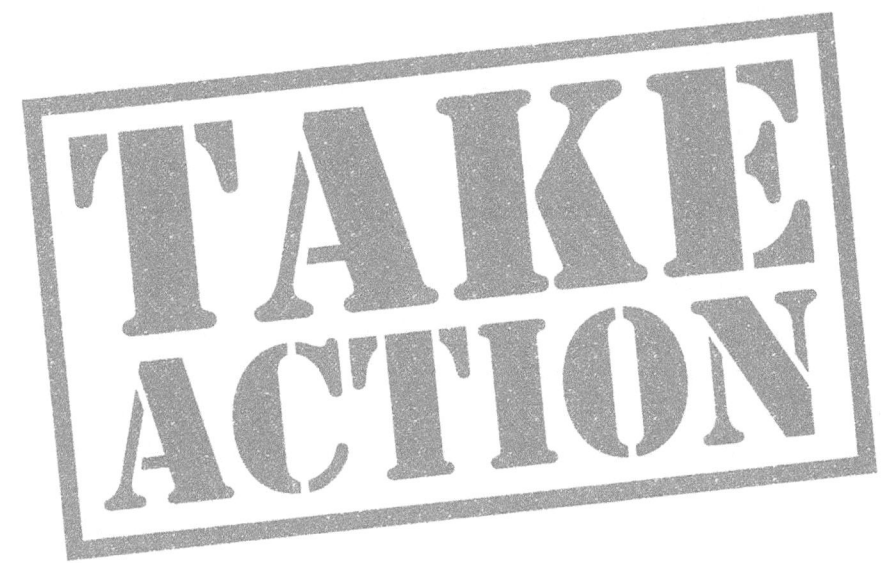

So you are ready to uncover your abs and you want to get started right away. The truth is there are a lot of variables when it comes to six pack ab training. It is best not to get in too much of a hurry, and to make sure all your bases are covered.

At the same time there is no time like the present to start working towards your fitness goals. Here are tips to get your started today towards the six pack you've always dreamed of.

Six Pack Action Plan

- Set Your Goal
- Set Your Timeline

- Structure Your Diet
- Decide on Checkpoints Along the Way
- Get Started

Set Your Goal – Ok we know your goal is a six pack, but you have to visualize exactly what that is. At what level will you be satisfied? You have to know how far you want to go before you decide on how you will get there. A good idea would be to find someone who's physique you admire and want to aspire to. Then cut it out or save it to your desktop and everyday spend a moment to look at it and visualize your body looking like that.

Set Your Timeline – You have to be realistic when it comes to how long it will take. Think about how long it took to gain all that extra weight in the first place. Get all those "8 weeks to abs" infomercials out of your head. You have to understand that getting a six pack, and then maintaining it is going to be a long term thing. If you set an unrealistic timeline you are likely to get frustrated and quit.

Structure Your Diet – We all know that most of the work for a six pack is done in the kitchen. You have to make sure that your diet is on point. More importantly you have to make sure it is right for you specifically. Just taking a diet off of a website won't guarantee success. You have to learn what foods, in what quantities work for you specifically.

Decide on Checkpoints Along the Way – Your long term goal is a six pack, but it is important to have planned checkpoints along the way. Whether it is weight loss or waist circumference you need to constantly monitor your progress to make sure you are on track. If you are not, then you need to change something.

Get Started – Don't wait around until everything is perfect. There never will be a perfect time to start. Just decide to start today. The more time you spend working towards your goal of a six pack the more you will learn about yourself. The best way to figure this all out is by doing. So don't put this off, and don't wait any longer. Clearly there is much more to ab training than this, but this is a good place to start. Everyone reacts differently to things and you will constantly have to monitor your progress to see what you need to change. One important thing, if what you are doing isn't working, change it. Don't keep doing the same thing over and over and expecting new results. At the same time don't change everything at once, or you won't know which change made the difference.

Well that brings us to an end of our beginners guide to revealing your six pack abs. I'm glad we've been able to take this journey towards six pack abs together, all the best with it and start today!

Meet the Author

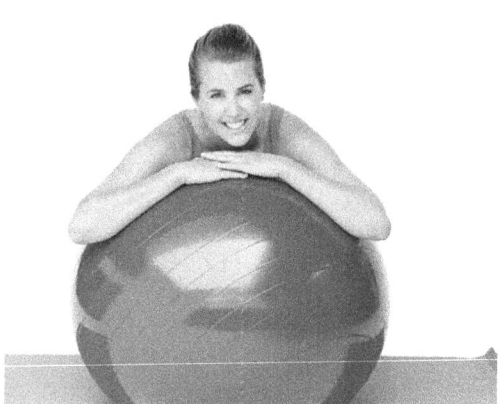

Certified personal trainer, nutrition and diet specialist and a wellness coach Kelly Larson's goal is to give as many people as possible the tools to start living a healthier lifestyle

Kelly believes that every person can achieve the body of their dreams through fitness, healthy eating and a balanced lifestyle. Kelly follows her own personal health and fitness philosophies and believes that a "perfect body" is not a realistic goal. The importance of good health should drive and motivate people to achieve better fitness and a better body. When you take care of your body as a whole you will start to feel better and your body will transform into looking better.

Kelly lives in sunny Florida and enjoys spending time with family and friends. Kelly is passionate about music, scuba diving and new adventures. In her spare time, Kelly volunteers at her local animal shelter.

More Books by Kelly Larson

Your Beach Body Transformation Begins Today: The Ultimate Guide to a Hot Summer Body

www.ingramcontent.com/pod-product-compliance
Ingram Content Group UK Ltd.
Pitfield, Milton Keynes, MK11 3LW, UK
UKHW050415240426
12048UKWH00020B/1522